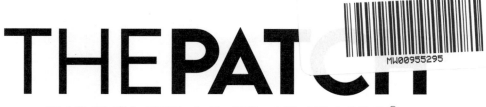

THEPATCH
DISCOVER LIVEWAVE X39®

©2024 HEALTH FREEDOM, LLC • PATCHEDU.COM
ISBN: 9798340455512

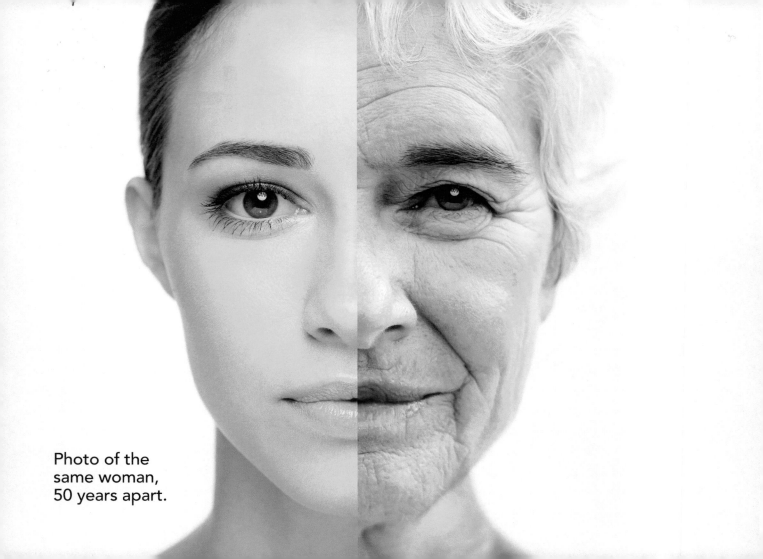

Photo of the
same woman,
50 years apart.

AGING PROCESS

As we age, our stem cells mutate and go dormant causing wrinkles, gray hair, body aches, and organ challenges. Many factors affect why mutations happen such as our genetic makeup, environmental factors, stress, lack of sleep, poor nutrition, and so on. Unhealthy stem cells circulating in our body is one of the main reasons we experience aging, discomfort, and disease.

Stem cells are special cells in the body that start out as a clean slate. These cells are called undifferentiated cells. This means stem cells can become any cell the body needs, such as heart cells, lung cells, skin cells, blood cells, or any other type of cell. Stem cells are necessary for healing and longevity. Having an abundance of healthy stem cells is key to aging well. The problem: healthy stem cells decline rapidly as we age.

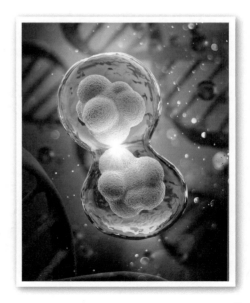

STEM CELL DETERIORATION
- **At age 20, we have a billion healthy stem cells**
- **By age 30, stem cells decline by 60% to 400 million**
- **By age 50, stem cells decline by 75% to 250 million**
- **By age 60, stem cells decline by 90% to 100 million**
- **By age 80, stem cells decline by 95% to 50 million**

PATENT

US 10,716,953 B1

X39 is "a wearable phototherapy apparatus that produces beneficial effects to a human body such as **activation of stem cells, improvement in strength, improvement in stamina, pain relief** via a non-transdermal container. The non-transdermal apparatus reflects or emits specific wavelengths of light to **elevate levels of the copper peptide GHK-CU in the body.**"

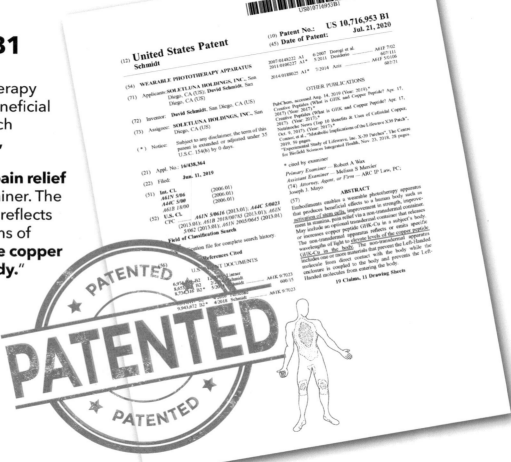

4

A double-blind test published in the "Internal Medicine Research - Open Journal" showed a significant increase in copper-peptide concentrations in the blood of subjects who had worn the X39 patches for only one week.

SOURCE: tinyurl.com/X39research

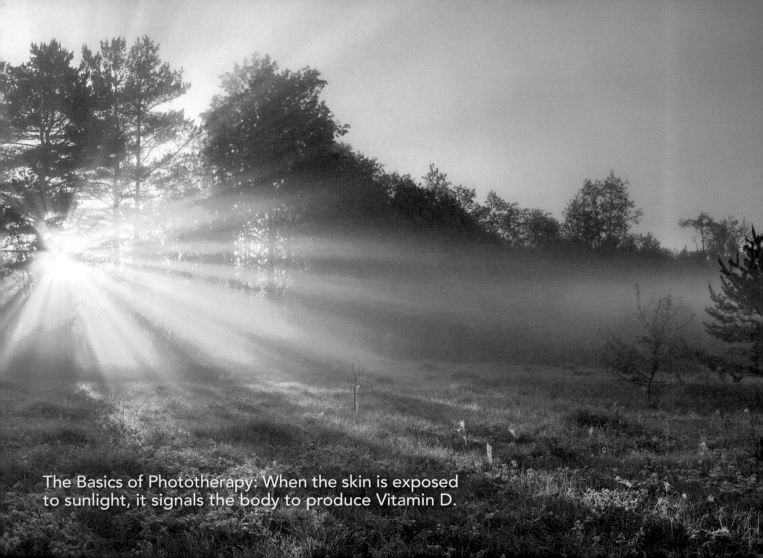

The Basics of Phototherapy: When the skin is exposed to sunlight, it signals the body to produce Vitamin D.

PHOTOTHERAPY

LifeWave patches use patented technology and work through a type of phototherapy called photobiomodulation. When applied to the skin, X39 reflects specific wavelengths of infrared light from your body onto the dermis of the skin, which then signals your body to increase specific peptide production. Another common example of phototherapy is when sunlight hits your skin, your body signals the production of vitamin D. The difference with X39 is that it uses your human infrared light.

GHK-CU AND MITOCHONDRIA

In the case of X39, it produces a copper peptide called GHK-Cu. As the dermis of the skin is stimulated by X39, mitochondria are activated, causing the body to produce more GHK-Cu. Mitochondria are involved in regulating the balance between the amount and quality of GHK-Cu that is produced. Mitochondria provide the necessary energy and metabolic support for human GHK-Cu production.

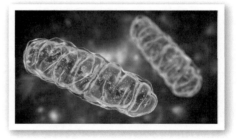

Mitochondria are responsible for generating most of the energy needed to power various cellular processes through cellular respiration. Cellular respiration is where mitochondria produce adenosine triphosphate (ATP), which serves as the energy currency of every cell. When your body is properly hydrated, along with getting the right electrolytes, mitochondria thrive and can greatly impact your body's ability to produce GHK-Cu.

PEPTIDES

Peptides are made up of a string of amino acids; anywhere from 2 to 50 different amino acids can form a peptide. Amino acids are essential for the structure and function of cells, tissues, and organs in the body, which is why they are often referred to as the building blocks of proteins.

X39 triggers GHK-Cu production in your body. GHK-Cu is a copper-bound tripeptide of glycine, histidine, and lysine. When you add copper from the body to GHK, you get an extremely important copper-bound tripeptide called GHK-Cu.

Binding copper to GHK tripeptide is how your body is able to increase healthy regenerative stem cell activity!

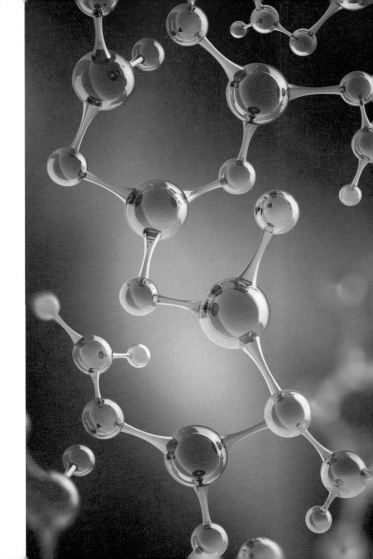

GHK-CU IS A COPPER-BOUND TRIPEPTIDE OF GLYCINE, HISTIDINE, AND LYSINE

GLYCINE

- Builds muscle
- Supports joint repair
- Produces collagen
- Reduces inflammation
- Protects the liver
- Protects the heart
- Improves metabolism
- Improves digestion
- Improves sleep quality

Deficiency Diseases:

Fatigue, breathing issues, weak muscle tone, seizures

HISTIDINE

- Supports growth
- Supports tissue repair
- Produces blood cells
- Protects nerve cells
- Produces histamine
- Supports immune function
- Supports digestion
- Improves sleep quality

Deficiency Diseases:

Anemia, slow wound healing, weak immune system, poor cognition, poor memory, stiff joints, arthritis

LYCINE

- Produces collagen
- Supports hormones
- Improves calcium levels
- Supports bone health
- Supports energy
- Improves immune system
- Helps block cortisol

Deficiency Diseases:

Fatigue, saggy skin, bone loss, agitation, anemia, nausea, loss of appetite, fatty-acid absorption issues, protein-energy deficiency

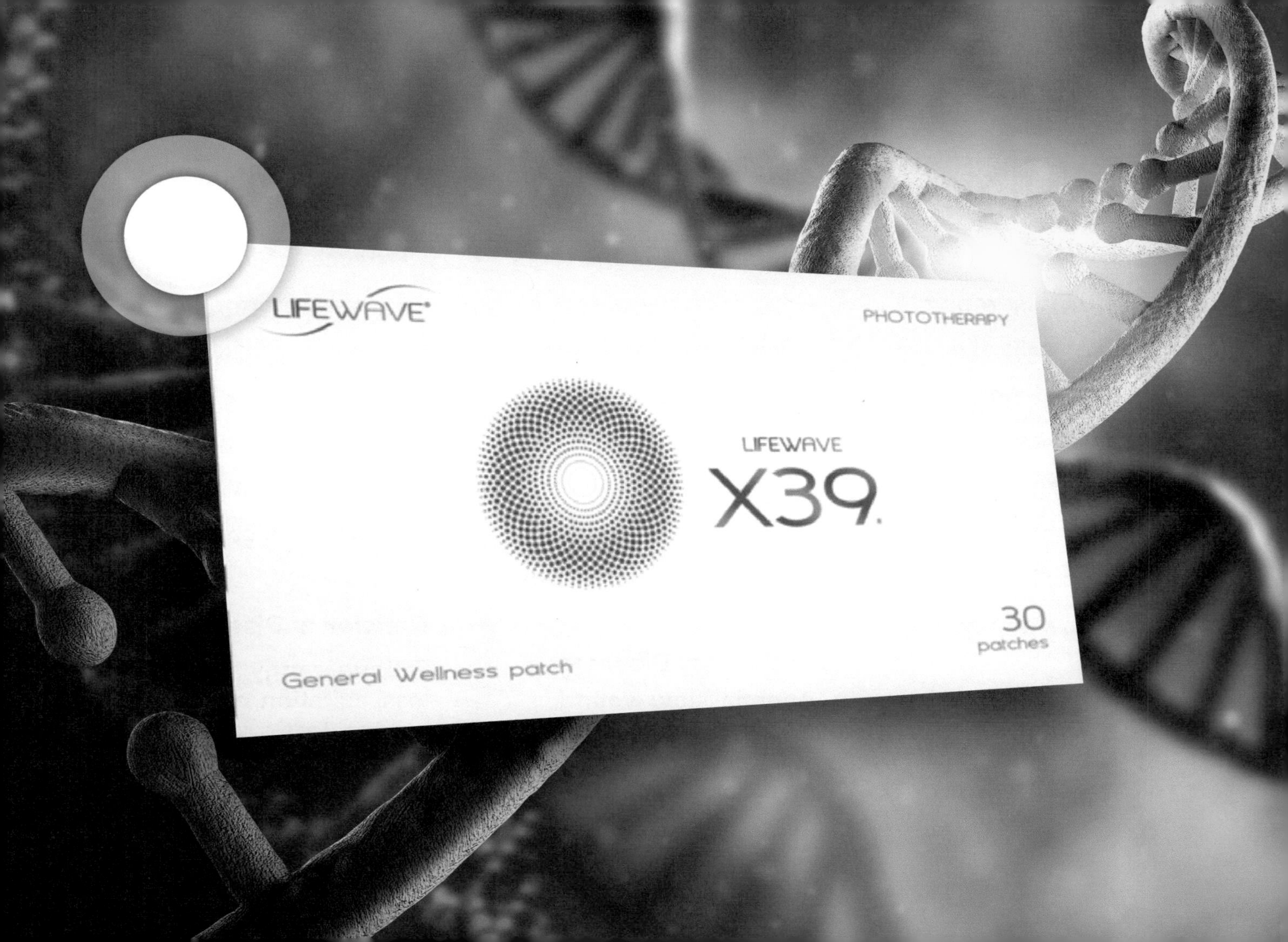
LIFEWAVE®
PHOTOTHERAPY
LIFEWAVE
X39.
30
patches
General Wellness patch

INFRARED LIGHT

X39 is a patented advanced technology that uses your body's own infrared light. Our bodies emit a form of infrared light that can be seen in thermal scans and with night vision goggles. This infrared light activates the patch causing it to reflect very specific wavelengths of light from the crystalline lattice pattern inside the patch back onto your skin. This low-light dermal activity from the X39 patch signals your body to produce specific peptides that then cause positive biochemical changes in the body.

The X39 patch is clinically proven to significantly increase human GHK-Cu copper peptide concentrations in the body, which increases healthy, youthful, regenerative stem cells. X39 is a safe, effective, and affordable way to reset 4,192 genes back to a healthier state.

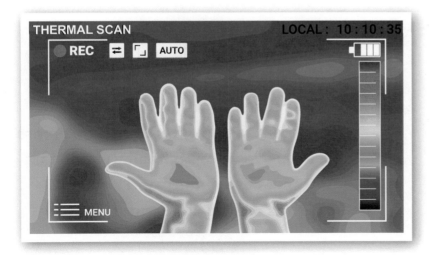

THERMAL SCAN   LOCAL : 10 : 10 : 35

● REC ⇄ ⌐ AUTO

☰ MENU

ABOUT LIFEWAVE X39 PATCHES

- FDA recognized and compliant "General Wellness Product"
- Made out of organic amino acids, salts, and sugars
- Non-transdermal
- Medical-grade plastic
- Hypoallergenic adhesive
- 96% effective rate
- Extremely affordable
- Patented technology
- No product in the world does what X39 does!

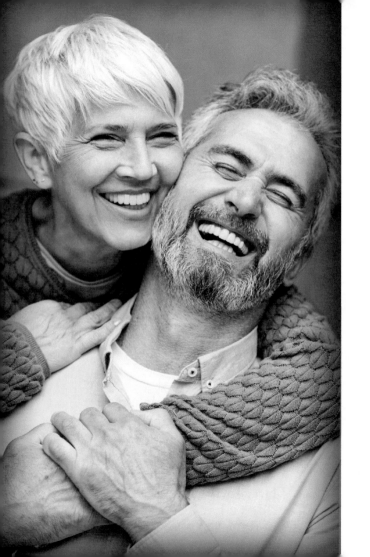

BENEFITS OF GHK-Cu COPPER PEPTIDE

A double-blind test that was published in the "Internal Medicine Research - Open Journal" showed there was a significant increase in GHK-Cu concentrations in the blood of subjects who had worn the X39 patches for only one week.

SOURCE: tinyurl.com/X39Research

Clinically proven to increase GHK-Cu copper peptide, which has the following benefits:

☑ **2,100% stem cell proliferation rate**

☑ **Works systemically - all over the body**

☑ **Reduces inflammation and pain**

☑ **Improves muscle and bone density**

☑ **Improves strength and stamina**

☑ **Increases collagen and elastin**

☑ **Increases hair growth and thickness**

☑ **Improves wound healing and scars**

☑ **Improves memory and clarity**

☑ **Eases anxiety and aggression**

BENEFITS OF X39

The X39 patch by LifeWave is the only patented technology available in the world that is clinically proven to increase healthy cells in the body. With a 96% efficacy rate, backed by gold-standard research and patents, your health is in good hands with LifeWave. Stay healthy with X39 today!

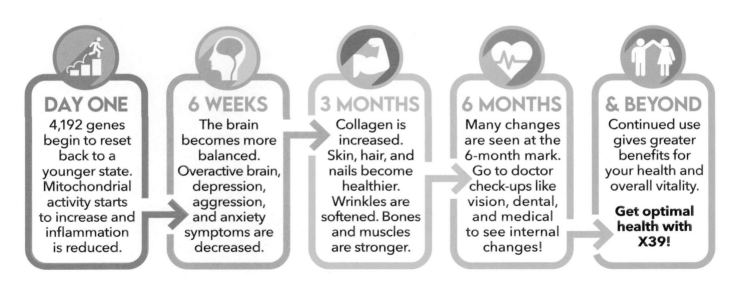

DAY ONE
4,192 genes begin to reset back to a younger state. Mitochondrial activity starts to increase and inflammation is reduced.

6 WEEKS
The brain becomes more balanced. Overactive brain, depression, aggression, and anxiety symptoms are decreased.

3 MONTHS
Collagen is increased. Skin, hair, and nails become healthier. Wrinkles are softened. Bones and muscles are stronger.

6 MONTHS
Many changes are seen at the 6-month mark. Go to doctor check-ups like vision, dental, and medical to see internal changes!

& BEYOND
Continued use gives greater benefits for your health and overall vitality.

Get optimal health with X39!

These statements have not been evaluated by the FDA. This product is not intended to treat, cure, or prevent any disease.

HOW TO USE X39

- Wear behind your neck, below your navel, or anywhere that needs extra attention

- Wear for 12 hours on and 12 hours off

- Repeat the next day with a new patch

- Drink plenty of water and consume good quality electrolytes daily

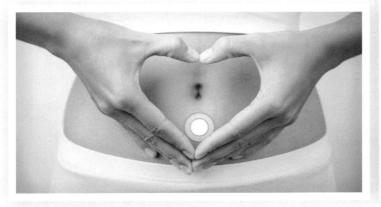

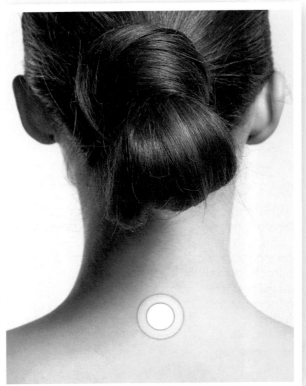

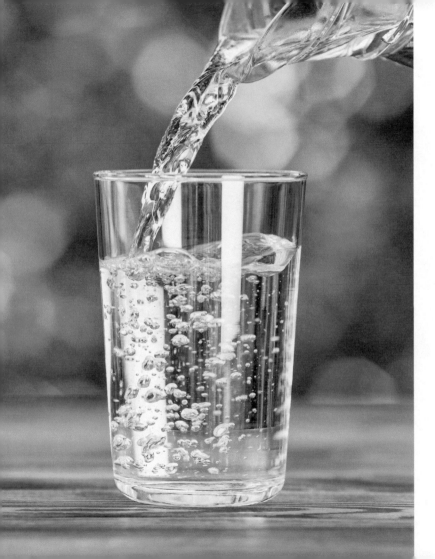

WHAT TO EXPECT

PERSONAL EXPECTATIONS
- Everyone responds differently
- Fill out the X39 Health Tracker
- Take note of specific issues
- Patches go to work where needed
- Internal healing may happen first
- Exhaustion is normal when healing
- If you are tired, it's working!
- Commit to 6-12 months
- Get normal doctor checkups

DETOXIFICATION SUPPORT
- Detox is common for 1-2 weeks
- Drink 4-5 ounces of water every 30 min. or a few sips every 15-20 min.
- Use a good electrolyte mix daily
- Limit or remove caffeine
- Get extra sleep, take naps
- Take an Epsom bath as needed
- Practice deep breathing

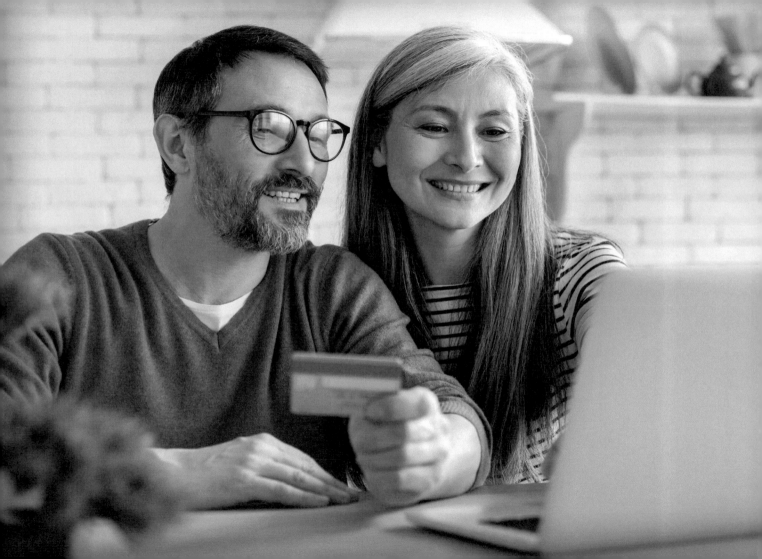

HOW TO ENROLL

STEPS TO ENROLL
- Go to www.LifeWave.com and enter your enroller's member number
- Make sure the name of the person you are enrolling with appears at the top
- Click JOIN and select a membership package – Core, Advanced, or Premium
- You get better discounts with larger packages
- Go through the steps, review your order, and click submit
- A final confirmation page with your member number will appear
- Check for confirmation emails from LifeWave for your order and subscription
- Contact your enroller to confirm you are signed up
- OPTIONAL: Fill out the Order Form on page 24 and your enroller will take a photo and get you enrolled with the best discount possible

BRAND PARTNER PACKAGES
The X39 patch is LifeWave's foundational health patch. Buying only X39 in your starter pack ensures you get the very best pricing. Adding Aeon can enhance the effectiveness of X39 when you have extra stress or inflammation. Choose the best pack for your needs!

- **Premium** - Best value at $1750 for 20 sleeves* of X39 or mix and match 40 credits**
- **Advanced** - Better value at $535 for 6 sleeves* of X39 or mix and match 12 credits**
- **Core** - Good value at $295 for 3 sleeves* of X39 or mix and match 6 credits**

   * Each sleeve contains 30 patches
   ** X39 and X49 count as two credits, while all other patch sleeves count as one

THE OPPORTUNITY

BENEFITS OF BECOMING A BRAND PARTNER
- Unique patented opportunity
- Professional Direct Sales
- Simple binary system - only two legs!
- Simple and effective building strategy
- Built-in onboarding system and training
- Earn while you learn opportunity
- Earn on Product Introductory Bonuses
- Earn on retail and customer accounts
- Earn up to $25,000 per week on Cycle Bonuses
- Earn 25% on Level 1 Cycle Bonuses
- Earn 20% on Level 2 and 3 Cycle Bonuses
- Unlimited earnings potential!

BASICS OF THE BINARY SYSTEM
- Only two legs to build
- Place people on your outside left and outside right only
- Get to Manager by sponsoring two people on each side
- Managers need 300 personal volume (PV) lifetime
- Managers need to be active at 110 personal volume (PV) per month
- Teach your personally sponsored to also rank to Manager
- Continue to build a strong team by teaching those under you to rank to Manager

Learn more about the opportunity with LifeWave at www.PatchEDU.com

Rank to Manager and teach others to rank to Manager!

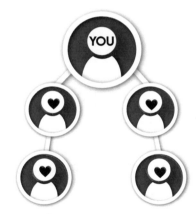

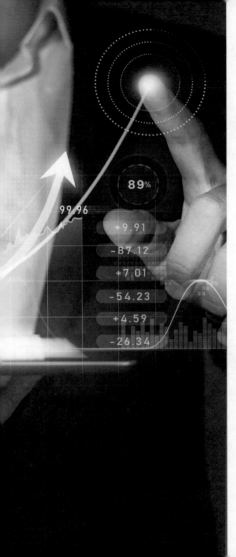

ABOUT LIFEWAVE

LIFEWAVE COMPANY STATISTICS
- Founded in 2004 by inventor, owner, and CEO David Schmidt
- Open in over 70 countries worldwide
- Innovative and patented products that no one else provides
- X39 launched in 2019 as the new foundational product
- X39 took 10 years and $4.5 million to develop
- Growth rate of 3,000% from 2018-2024
- From $20 million to over $600 million annually in five years
- The fastest growing network marketing company in the world
- Winner of the 2024 Direct Selling News Bravo Growth Award
- 9th largest growth rate direct sales company in the world
- Ranked 32 on DSN Global 100 list based on revenue in 2023

DAVID SCHMIDT STATISTICS
- Scientist, inventor, founder, and CEO
- Holds over 150 patents
- Over 80 clinical trials on the patches
- Honorary Doctor of Science and Technology
- Two-time recipient of the Advanced Technology
  Award from the International Hall of Fame

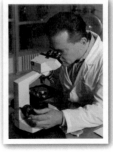

LIFEWAVE INCOME DISCLOSURE

RANK	Percent of active Brand Partners	2023 Annual Earnings for Active Brand Partners			Average Months to Achieve Rank*
		HIGH	LOW	AVERAGE	
BRAND PARTNER	93%	$30,329	$3	**$40**	–
MANAGER	6%	$74,490	$5	**$1,709**	4
DIRECTOR	1%	$111,703	$15	**$8,217**	8
SENIOR DIRECTOR	<1%	$67,267**	$50	**$16,248**	10
EXECUTIVE DIRECTOR	<1%	$121,430	$500	**$45,677**	15
PRESIDENTIAL DIRECTOR	<1%	$203,896	$14,309	**$79,806**	16
SENIOR PRES. DIRECTOR	<1%	$2M+	$2,286	**$396,580**	24

* Measured from the date of enrollment. ** The number for Senior Director in the "HIGH" category is correct as it is based on the highest individual payout for that rank in 2023. High means the highest any one person in that rank category was paid, low means the lowest any one person in that rank category was paid, and average is what the total average was paid for all people in that rank.

INCOME POTENTIAL

The average time it takes to get to Senior Presidential Director is only two years of full time work! **What would you do with an extra $396,580 per year?**

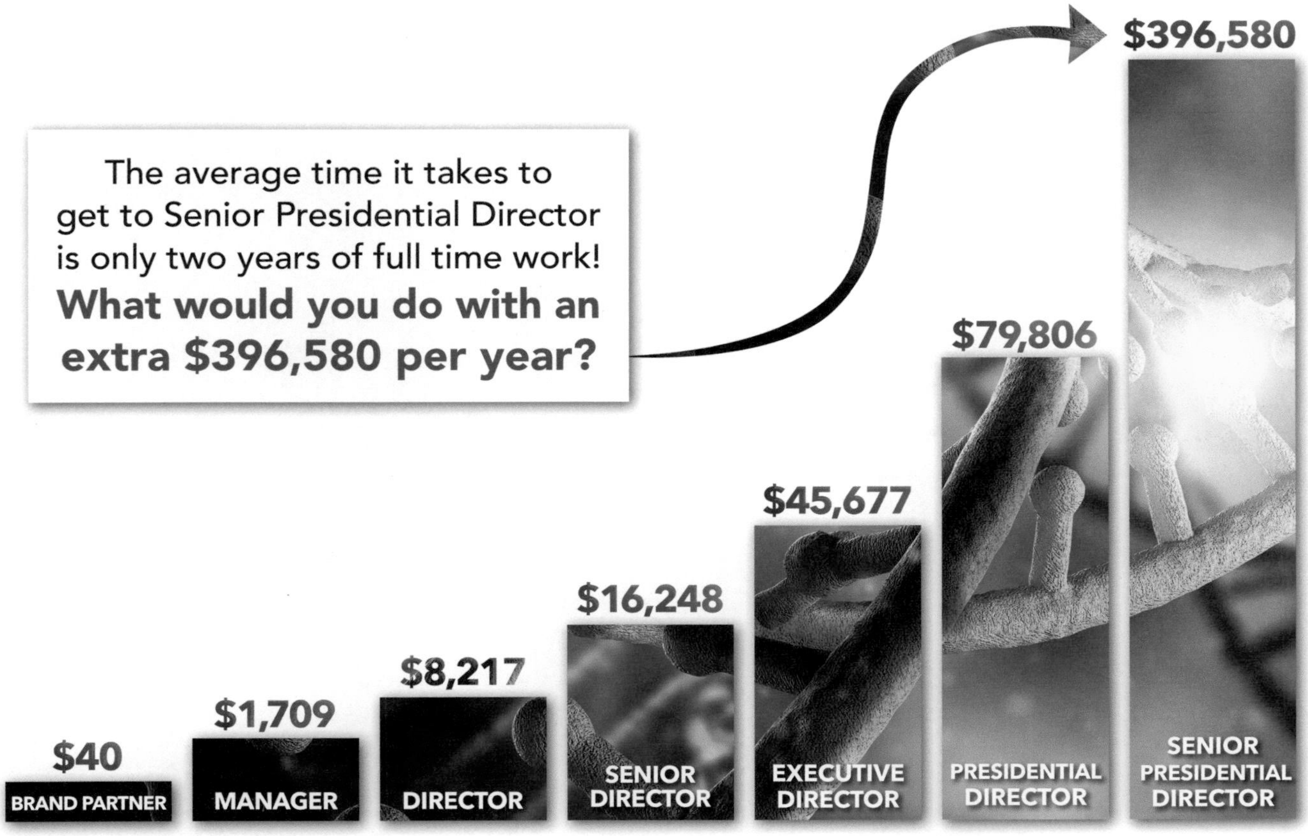

$396,580

$79,806

$45,677

$16,248

$8,217

$1,709

$40

BRAND PARTNER | **MANAGER** | **DIRECTOR** | **SENIOR DIRECTOR** | **EXECUTIVE DIRECTOR** | **PRESIDENTIAL DIRECTOR** | **SENIOR PRESIDENTIAL DIRECTOR**

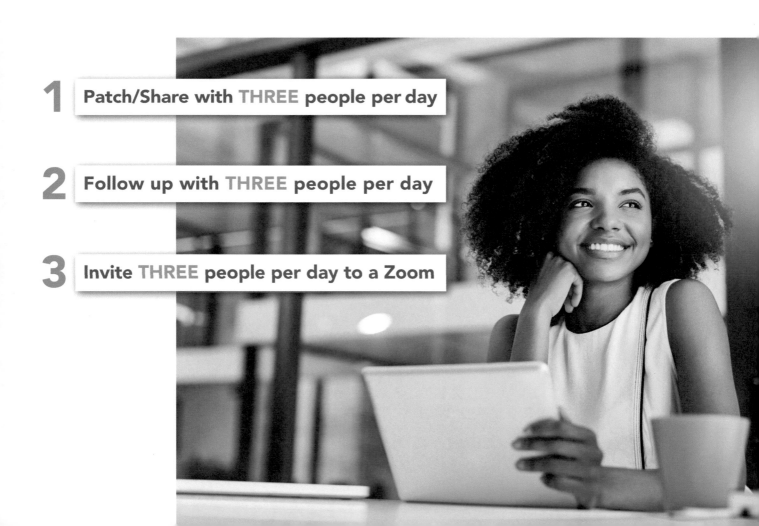

1 Patch/Share with THREE people per day

2 Follow up with THREE people per day

3 Invite THREE people per day to a Zoom

THE 3-STEP SYSTEM

STEP ONE – Patch 3
Physically put one X39 patch on **three** new people per day or share PatchEDU.com with **three** new people per day online. Only share X39 for maximum growth potential. For online people, simply ask your friend to watch the first two short videos on PatchEDU.com. A great way to introduce X39 is to send a 30-60 second voice text with passion and excitement in your voice. "Hey (name)! I am having amazing success with a new technology that I know you will want to try for you and your family! Do you have five minutes to watch a very short video? I would really appreciate your thoughts on this. Let me know and I hope you are well!" Then follow up with step two.

STEP TWO – Follow up with 3
Follow up with **three** people per day. Follow up examples:
> "Watch the first two short videos on PatchEDU.com"
> "Do you have stress and inflammation?"
> "Are you interested in a side hustle?"
> "Check out this video about X39." Choose a short YouTube video about X39.

STEP THREE – Invite 3
Invite **three** people per day to a Zoom that also shares the opportunity.
- Invite each person to two different Zoom times to give them options.
- Attend with them and get them involved either via text or on the chat on Zoom.
- Go over the income disclosure with them after the event. See page 20-21.

BASIC LIFEWAVE ORDER FORM

**EACH SLEEVE CONTAINS 30 PATCHES • APPLY PATCHES TO CLEAN, DRY SKIN AND WEAR FOR 12 HOURS. WEAR A NEW PATCH DAILY.
POINTS ARE FOR BIANARY COMPENSATION • X39 AND X49 COUNT AS 2 CREDITS, WHILE ALL OTHER PATCH SLEEVES COUNT AS ONE**

PREMIUM
☐
FOR LARGE FAMILIES
OR THE SERIOUS ENTREPRENEUR
$1750 USD
THREE MONTHS ACTIVE STATUS
30-DAY GUARANTEE
(745 POINTS)
20 SLEEVES X39
40 CREDITS

ADVANCED
☐
FOR MEDIUM SIZED FAMILIES
OR THE NEW BUSINESS BUILDER
$535 USD
30-DAY GUARANTEE
(300 POINTS)
6 SLEEVES X39
12 CREDITS

CORE
☐
FOR INDIVIDUALS & COUPLES
OR TO GET STARTED SLOWER
$295 USD
30-DAY GUARANTEE
(180 POINTS)
3 SLEEVES X39
6 CREDITS

SUBSCRIPTION OPTIONS
☐ **TWO SLEEVES OF X39**
$199⁹⁰ USD PER MONTH (154 PV)

☐ **X39/X49 PERFORMANCE PACK**
$179⁹⁵ USD PER MONTH (140 PV)

☐ **ONE SLEEVE OF X39**
$99⁹⁵ USD PER MONTH (77 PV)

☐ **ONE SLEEVE OF AEON**
$69⁹⁵ USD PER MONTH (55 PV)

MEMBER INFORMATION

FIRST AND LAST NAME

MOBILE PHONE

ADDRESS

EMAIL

CITY, STATE, ZIP

DATE OF BIRTH

YOUR DESIRED USER NAME
LifeWave.com/

PASSWORD

SPONSOR'S NAME OR ID NUMBER

PAYMENT INFORMATION

☐ BILLING ADDRESS SAME AS SHIPPING

NAME ON CREDIT CARD

BILLING ADDRESS IF DIFFERENT THAN ABOVE

CARD NUMBER

EXPIRATION MONTH/YEAR

CVV CODE

SIGNATURE

DATE

Made in United States
Troutdale, OR
10/30/2024